Quinoa Cookbook Journey

21 *Shockingly Delicious Recipes* to
Honor the Taste Buds and the Body

Featuring Traditional & Not So Traditional Holiday
Recipes, Comfort Food Casseroles & Delectable Desserts

From the Creator of
foodRevelation.com
and "Food *IS* Talking"

Intuitive Chef Gail Blair

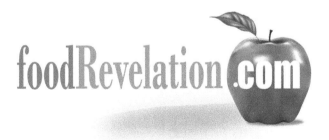

All Recipes are Gluten Free, Vegetarian with **Vegan** Options

Quinoa Cookbook Journey
By Gail Blair
Copyright 2016

The information in this book and related material in the form of tips, recipes, and nutritional guidance does not qualify as a substitution for your medical doctor's advice. Seek guidance from your doctor concerning your health and wellness; in particularly with respect to any symptoms that may require diagnosis or medical attention.

Printed in the United States of America
First Printing 2016
ISBN: 978-0-692-80181-9
EFH Publishing
For more info or bulk ordering visit http://foodrevelation.com/ or call 214-770-1925

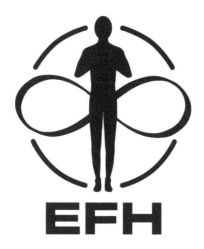

EFH

At first glance this book may look like your typical cookbook (if you consider quinoa typical). I assure you it is not. What makes this cookbook unique? It was written by a very creative, Plant-Based Chef turned *"Food and Medical Intuitive"*. How creative? Intuitive Chef Gail Blair has been lovingly labeled, the **plant-based chef for "Meat-Lovers" and "Vegetable Haters"**. Her recipes surprise and amaze even the most skeptical, die-hard meat and potato lover, including me. The bonus of her "intuitive gift" is a gift that keeps on giving. If you think "healthy" means suffering through tasteless, cardboard box meals, you are in for a big treat! There is a divine reason Gail was a master chef before her "gifts" kicked in. No-one wants to suffer on the road to health. As a client, I can attest with Gail you don't have to.

- John Sklar M.D./Pain Specialist and creator of Pathways to Releasing Pain

For years I've tried every diet in the book, lose some weight without enjoying food and then gain it right back. Gail's Food Compatibility Consultation was an eye opener. For the first time I now understand what specific foods my body needs to be healthy. I was able to bring my body into balance within 10 days. The bonus was losing 10 pounds exactly where I wanted to lose them while eating as much as I wanted with the foods compatible for my body. Gail is a genius at creating recipes that are delicious, easy to make and family friendly. I can't say enough about how freeing it is to finally understand what I need for my body. The fun part is that Gail's intuitive approach along with a great big helping of common sense is served with a side of humor.

- Marie Guthrie/CEO – Executive Leadership Strategist – Quantum Leader Foundation Program

In Love, Appreciation and Gratitude...

I dedicate this book to the Universe. I am so grateful for your never-ending support of my dreams. Thank you! Thank you! Thank you! To my precious granddaughter Jadyn; my amazing children Jackie, Justin and Jerett, who have all helped raise me.

A shout out to some wonderful folks who agreed to test drive and critique all the recipes. Their feedback was priceless! I am so grateful to Marie Guthrie for supplying the inspiration that started this ball rolling; your cooking skills and expert taste buds! Big thanks to your entire family for being my guinea pigs.

Thank you Dr. John Sklar for your bravery, feedback, support and amazing endorsement!

It is impossible to describe the immense gratitude I feel for my family and friends for your open mind and acceptance of all my "weird ways".

To Alida Morrill/Balance Your Life. You are an amazing energy coach, friend and mentor; I may have gotten this far without you, but it would not have been this easy and I'm so grateful I didn't have to. Bless you for saving me from "myself" too many times to count.

Huge hugs of gratitude to Allison Fields of Big Iki Coaching for helping me remove blocks to finishing this project and become a better, "lighter" writer. And, for your proofing and editing skills!

Kristen Vega – Photographer/Designer. Your help has been priceless! Thank you for the tireless hours you spent with me cooking and your unique intuitive skill; helping me hit one recipe Home Run after another. I am so grateful for your eye for detail that resulted in mouth-watering photos.

Chris Alcocer – Thank you for your expert photo editing. You took the amazing and made it incredible!

And, last but definitely not least; to all my clients who unwittingly became taste-testers as I have shared these recipes with you all along as part of the "**Food _IS_ Talking**" journey. Thank you for all of your praise and support. It is the work with you that blesses my days. I am grateful and I love you!

Table of Contents

Introduction

Hi there! This is Intuitive Chef Gail Blair, coming to you from a little town in the heart of North Texas. I never dreamed I would be writing a quinoa cookbook! Heck, 10 years ago I didn't even know what quinoa was! If anyone had told me 5 years ago where my passion for cooking and love for food would lead me, I would have said that someone is CRAAAZZZY!

This passion led me on a journey of self-discovery and along the way I found my true calling: helping others discover for themselves their natural health and "intuitive" gifts. Yes, health is natural – *chronic disease is not.*

Why is Quinoa the star of this cookbook? It is a complete protein (like meat and dairy); making it a vegan's best friend and perfect for anyone looking to reduce their meat intake. AND, it is easily digested, low glycemic, nutrient dense, and alkaline to neutral in pH. It cooks in as little as 15 minutes and freezes perfectly. It also happens to be super versatile! Having very little flavor on its own, it's like a painter's blank canvas just waiting to be painted. So that's what I've done! Created Quinoa Art!

As you cook your way through this little book, enjoying every blissful bite, you will be learning how to create balance in the body. As in all of life and nature, balance is crucial to flourishing health.

You will find enclosed a surprisingly delicious collection of traditional casseroles, side dishes and desserts; along with some very creative, natural ways to enjoy full-flavor food without punishing the taste buds. Many recipes are re-vamped holiday traditions. Each one has been test-driven by the most discerning foodies across the U.S.

My Motto - *"The taste buds don't care if the food is plant, animal or healthy as long as it's delicious!"*

Most of the recipes in this little book are simple and designed for families to cook and enjoy together. Some a little more challenging, but easy to follow. Who doesn't like a fun, delicious challenge? Many are "all-in-one" meals. I knew you wanted to hear that! All of them are **gluten-free, vegetarian and/or vegan friendly**. And, most of them freeze very well; so even the single person or small family can enjoy the luxury of having something healthful and delicious every day!

This book is also the natural result of over 400 **"Intuitive Food Compatibility Sessions"** over almost 5 years now. It is an accumulation of what has been revealed intuitively (revelation) and learned along the way through experience. Three common threads run through most sessions:

1. Many bodies are "malnourished" (obesity is a primary symptom of this – YES);
2. Many bodies are "unbalanced" (too acidic – at the root of all chronic disease) and
3. Many bodies are "over-proteinated" (a new word that means the body is getting WAY too much protein from mostly acidic sources).

The delicious recipes contained within are rich in "alkaline forming foods". What does this mean? All foods have a pH level and affect the pH of the body once processed by the body. (Here is a fun little site that explains what pH is: http://chemistry.about.com/od/ph/f/What-Does-Ph-Stand-For.htm).

A pH of 7.0 is neutral (foods that are neutral do not affect the pH of the body). A pH below 7.0 is acidic and above 7.0 is alkaline. **Wrap your head around this:** Acid burns (inflames) flesh inside and out. Eating too much acidic food leads to inflammation in the body and this chronic inflammation leads to chronic disease.

Optimum body pH matches the blood pH*. To support life, the blood pH must be maintained between 7.35 – 7.45. (A body pH over 7.0 supports health). Some may say what we eat doesn't affect the pH. It may not affect the blood pH for a long time; however, the body is constantly striving to keep the crucial narrow blood pH within a life-supporting range; until it can't anymore. At that point the body has been robbed of health, trying to maintain life at all cost. The cost is a slow decaying (dying) body.

The "body's ability" to maintain "life supporting" blood pH is MOST CERTAINLY affected by what we eat. A blood pH outside of the life-supporting narrow range confirms the body is really sick. (By the way, I'm talking about over-all body pH, not organ pH - they vary*).

You can know before the body becomes sick when it is struggling to maintain optimum blood pH simply by keeping track of body pH. This is true "prevention"! The most accurate way to test your body pH is with a litmus strip and your saliva. I've found between lunch and dinner (3 hours after eating or drinking anything) is the best time, based on the numbers I receive intuitively. Be sure to spit a couple of times to clear the mouth of any interference.

The body is either in "thriving" mode or "decaying" mode;
there is no in between.
What we eat and think determines the mode.

I don't know about you, but I want to be in "thriving" mode.

The recipes in this book are "mostly" neutral, alkaline forming or very low acidic (see the **Chart of Foods**). As you eat your way through this unique cookbook, you will be satisfying your taste buds and providing your body with a "reasonable" amount of easy to digest, "body balancing" protein.

I'm going to help you keep the balance by providing the **"Chart of Foods"** (that started it all) at the end of this book. Our bodies need alkaline and acidic food. They just need more alkaline than acidic. The chart will help you know what's what.

Once the body has achieved balance it is easy to maintain. There will be no need for deprivation or strict dieting. You can eat anything as long as it is real (nature-made) food and still maintain balance, when you know how to create it.

It DOES matter what we eat. However, what is even more important is what we *THINK*. It doesn't matter much what we eat if our thoughts are toxic. Stress creates excess acid in the body making it very hard if not impossible to maintain healthy balance.

The high vibration of abundant health is not compatible
with the energy of unhappiness or stress.

I share ALL the revelations I've received since 2012 (when the "Intuitive Chef" journey began) in the upcoming book **"Evolution of FREE Health"** – *The 6 Missing Links to Abundant Health.*

For more on **"Intuitive Food Compatibility Testing"** go to: http://foodrevelation.com/.

These "Intuitive Food Compatibility Sessions" (I call it "Food *IS* Talking") also reveal that people have A LOT of digestive issues and food intolerances. And, many are way out of balance. What the body cannot digest it cannot use. What the body cannot use becomes a big burden to the body.

> NO "Good" food is good for every "body" all the time, no matter how healthy or balanced it may be.

Quinoa is one of the foods that testing consistently compatible to most clients **(There are others – Stay tuned for** "Food *IS* Talking" **The 10 Most Compatible Foods Cookbook").**

This amazing "grain-like" seed is neutral to alkaline in pH (helps balance an over-acidic body). Amaranth is another amazing seed with these qualities; however, quinoa has proven over time with my clients to be more compatible with more people.

> A balanced body is a healthy body!

Here's the short story of how I arrived at this place in my life, writing The Quinoa Cookbook Journey (the long story is told in **"Evolution of FREE Health" - coming soon**). It has been quite a ride!

Back in 2009, I was asking myself , *"What are you going to do Gail with the rest of your life?".* I was in my early 50's, had raised 3 children as a single mom (still single) and was currently bartending. Fine Dine bartending served me very well in times of transition, but I couldn't see doing it much longer. I've done a lot of things in my life and I've never been afraid of change. Little did I know, I was in for a BIG ONE!

I only had 3 criteria at that point. This new career had to be something I loved that didn't feel like work; it had to serve others and it had to take me through retirement. That was all – pretty wide open!

I was reading one of those so-called "self-help" books one day (I don't recall the title). The book was a "how to" guide in discovering your passion to uncover your purpose. The only thing I do remember about the book was this; if you start working your passion, your purpose will naturally show up. The trick was to think back when you were about 12 and recall what lit you up. What from your childhood remains a passion?

I was so passionate about reading – still am! The world around me stops when my head is stuck in a good book. I prefer reading to TV. My kids joke the addiction to books was the cause of my divorce (NOT). This passion has been leading me to writing all along, but I didn't see that then.

I loved sketching horses, but hadn't drawn since I was a teenager until just recently. The only other passion from my childhood that has been consistent throughout my life is my love for food and cooking. I decided that was it!

I was having fun cooking with my Dad for a family of 7 by the time I was 12. My Dad is a fantastic chef! He always says to me, *"You're a chip off the ole block!"*. Over the years I've learned to cook all types of cuisines; some before the age of the internet. I have a natural gift for discerning flavors and combining spices. Creating recipes is one of my favorite past times! It's like scoring a home run when one turns out perfect the first time at bat! My intuitive skills have helped me hit a lot of home runs!

As an evolving vegan (evolution happens slowly); revamping traditional holiday recipes into new healthy traditions became an obsession. Daddy still can't figure out why he doesn't miss the meat in my soups and chili. I share many of my secrets on Facebook at https://www.facebook.com/foodrevelation/ and on WordPress at https://foodistalking.wordpress.com/

Several recipes in this book have made their home at our family's holiday table: Sweet Corn Casserole (my dad's favorite), Holiday Green Bean Casserole and Decadent & Dark Quinoa Brownies. The carrot cake in this book will be next. It already has my dad's stamp of approval.

Okay – Back to the journey. I was so excited to get started working my passion, I immediately hooked up with a friend and we began catering within a couple of short months. It didn't take long to realize catering wasn't exactly it. Way too much stress and not enough income were zapping my joy. After about a year, I closed the door on that business. As with all "perceived" failure, I learned some valuable lessons and had some amazing experiences. **What I learned:**

1. Don't jump into something before giving it sufficient time to percolate.
2. If something doesn't flow easily and bring you joy, then you might be barking up the wrong tree. When you are in the flow (or zone as some call it) you can work endlessly and tirelessly.
3. When a door slams shut, don't keep trying to open it!

One of my favorite experiences: My business partner (a very talented "Paula Deen style" chef) and I developed a series of cooking classes called "Dueling Chefs" for a large local book store. We went "toe to toe" every other week, creating our own versions of Southern holiday recipes. The audience voted on their favorite. Much to my surprise, I won many of these duels and became known locally as *"The Plant-based Chef for "Meat Lovers" and "Vegetable Haters"*

As the door closed on catering, foodRevelation.com rolled in right away like a refreshing breeze. I had no idea how ***"relevant"*** the name would be at the time. My life was about to change drastically! My purpose was unfolding. This journey has revealed one revelation after another!

foodRevelation.com began on this simple premise, ***"We have been provided the perfect tool kit for optimum health AND it comes from one of the greatest pleasures on Earth – FOOD. Glorious Food!"*** I believed Hippocrates was correct when he quipped, *"Let food be thy Medicine and Medicine be thy food".*

My main focus was teaching others how to cook delicious, plant-based food everyone loves – even meat lovers. I stayed busy with cooking classes and demos at venues such as; Le Creuset, Market

Street Grocers, wellness centers; for individuals and small private parties.

During this time I started volunteering at my local food bank. I was helped there as a client at a very lean time in my life. I will be forever grateful! This relationship led to the extreme honor of sitting on the committee whose goal was to convert this pantry into a real *"Nutrition Center"*. This amazing "one of kind" pantry supplies organic produce and whole foods to the ones who need it most, while honoring the unique diet needs of every client. Vegans, Vegetarians and those with health challenges like diabetes, heart disease, gluten intolerance, etc. can find real nourishment here. My dream is to see this model spread across Texas and beyond.

I also worked as a private chef for a family of 4, responsible for creating and preparing meals compatible with their very strict **"anti-fungal"** diet. This family was not looking forward to 9 to 12 months of boring food. The Universe put us together and I was hired at our first meeting. This "anti-fungal" diet experience was the catalyst for "Food *IS* Talking" **Intuitive Food Compatibility Testing** that helped "fast-track" this diet journey.

"Gail is an AMAZING chef. The way that she can take healthy foods and put them all together to make an exquisite meal is amazing. Our dietary requirements were very limited (no dairy, grains or sugar) and when Gail cooked for us we felt like there was not a thing missing from our diets". - Staci Wright

As my gifts evolved and expanded, a whole new world opened up! This health food junkie and "miss know-it-all" had to eat some humble pie as this revelation rolled in, "**Not one good food is good for every "body" all of the time**. It's not about what is good or bad, only about what is compatible. Every "body" is completely unique.

What the "body" needs for optimum health changes according to what is going on physically, mentally and even spiritually; even by what we ate the day before and even as we heal. Oh, and not one so-called "Bad Food" is bad for everyone either (as long as it is *"real food"*). I realized as well, our natural, organic bodies are only compatible with natural, real food. Not chemicals.

Long story short, "Food *IS* Talking" was born and new ways to serve others became clear. We have the ability to know what is compatible to our bodies at any given time. In addition to cooking classes, I started sharing with others **how** *"food is talking"* and what it's saying through private sessions and workshops.

The next big revelation - **Not only are our bodies a reflection of what we eat; but more importantly, what we "*Think*".** Our thoughts affect our health and our life. Health and unhappiness cannot co-exist together for very long. The revelations continue...

The inspiration for this book came from another recipe, as so often happens. My client (became best friend) who is also a huge foodie and I were hanging out, preparing breakfast one beautiful spring morning. Her "certified" nature preserve that happens to be her backyard inspires inspiration! She made this quinoa thingy the night before from a recipe she had found online (Gabby's Gluten Free). It was like a spongy sweet bread; really delicious and simple!

I was thinking out loud and said, "Wow! I could do a lot with this!" Marie said, "How about a quinoa recipe cookbook?" Within the next 30 minutes we had decided on a book of 30 recipes (reduced to 21 in the end) and already we had 12 ideas. When something flows in that easily, you are in the zone! It has been a joy and a breeze to write this book. Other cookbooks are in the pipeline so stay tuned!

All of the recipes in this book contain a healthy amount of easy to digest, whole protein per serving. One cup of cooked quinoa alone provides 8 grams of whole protein.

It's important to get the required protein your body needs, but it is just as important not to go overboard. Too much protein is hard on the body, particularly the kidneys.
http://www.huffingtonpost.com/2014/06/12/eating-too-much-protein_n_5481307.html/

Every "body" is different and protein needs change. However, according to the CDC (by the way you can no longer access this information) the average female needs 45 grams of protein a day and the average male 55. (This is in line with what I get intuitively). If you are a meat-eater, following the USDA guidelines you will consume on average 88 grams of protein a day; way too much protein for most people.

How does this happen? Most plant food has protein and some plants, like quinoa, kale and lentils, to name a few; provide whole protein (just like meat). Our body has a requirement for the amino acids that make up a whole protein. However, not all protein has all essential amino acids (amino acids your body doesn't make). It is easy to achieve your protein requirement by just eating a variety of foods. Yes, variety is the spice of life! (This became really clear in repeated **Intuitive Food Compatibility Sessions overtime**

with clients).

I have realized through these sessions that some people REALLY DO need meat (just not in the large quantities Americans have been consuming over the last 50 years or so). However, for the sake of creating balance (this book is about that), I have not included any. Feel free to add a little meat if your body is screaming for it and be sure to balance it with plenty of green veggies. A good rule to follow is 2 servings of veggies with a 4 ounce serving of meat. (I share "alkalizing" salad dressings in the **"Before We Get Started"** section).

You may be ready for change, but just a little worried the change won't taste good. You may have bought the idea that healthy cannot possibly be "taste bud" worthy. This is a myth and just not true; as many of my clients, friends and family can attest!

You may have gotten out of the habit of giving your food and your body the attention and love they deserve. When we love, honor and respect our body it loves us back with good health. And, love makes everything taste better! A lot of love went into creating every recipe. Each creation celebrates food - glorious food! And, the miracle of it to bless our bodies with health!

Wishing you all Peace, Joy, LOVE & Health!

Intuitive Chef Gail

What Clients Are Saying About
Intuitive Chef Gail Blair...

"The time I spent with Gail learning about the Intuitive process and energy was worth every moment of my time, and time should be taken very seriously. It wasn't simply something to hear it was a skill that she is great at teaching and I can carry it out in my daily journey to reach my Self goals and continue to become a healthier, happier me. The incredible recipes she has created and shared have changed my outlook on what "healthy" can taste like. Aside from her cooking and teaching, her energy and attitude are so contagious. I'm glad that through this journey we have become friends and we can share questions, thoughts and ideas with each other. She not only worked with my Mother (to improve her health) and me, but she also worked with my horses and taught me things about them that will make our relationship stronger as well. I can't say enough about how beneficial meeting Gail at that time in my journey as been!"
Johnny Hogan/Ardmore, OK

"WOW! All I can say is that every single recipe that I've tried has been delicious! You are an amazing chef! My hubby wanted to take the Curry Red Lentil soup to work to have his Indian Coworker try it because it was that good. He said it was restaurant quality and to keep it in our rotation of recipes. My daughter (11yrs old)) asked for me to puree it and she loved it too. Made the Ranch Dressing and my daughter raved about it. So, thank you for making this part not so difficult and oh so fabulously delicious!"
Penny Berman/Richardson, TX

"I thank God often for bringing Chef Gail Blair into my life. I started seeing her for intuitive food compatibility testing about 10 months ago. I had been very sick for months. I saw several doctors and even a holistic doctor 2000 miles away. I was afraid to look in the mirror at my frail reflection and eating wasn't often a comfortable experience.

Her intuitive food charts took the guess work out of eating. I focused on the foods my body needed and was quickly needing a new chart with exciting new foods on it that I'd hadn't dreamed were part of my natural diet. I committed to the healing process, no matter what ideas I'd held about the surprises on the chart. Dairy and coffee took a leap of faith, but I love them both now. I am back up to a healthy weight and I LOVE food!

I have had the unique opportunity to have sampled a lot of Chef Gail's cooking. Her food is amazing! She loves what she does and you can taste it in her meals. I love everything I've had so far and I can't wait to see what comes next!"
Kristen Vega/Richardson, TX

"I was very impressed at how good the food tasted for "vegan". I've tasted some vegan products before and was not impressed. The root vegetable and lentil soup was awesome and the cornbread divine! I ate every morsel. The chili had a great kick and you would never know there was no meat in it. It tasted delicious. The sweet potato pie was yummy! I can't wait to try these recipes on my family next. I would definitely recommend anyone to try these recipes. It was all very YUMMY. I am a believer now that healthy CAN taste WONDERFUL. Gail, those recipes ROCK!!!"
Martina Chamberlain/ From Market Street Cooking Class "Down Home Roots"

"Gail Blair you are amazing!! Thank you so much for such an extraordinary session today. I feel confident and validated in the food choices I will be making. I have been praying for someone like you to come into my life and here you are!! I gained so much information and understanding about what is going on with me physically and spiritually. You are so comprehensive and thorough that I felt so completely empowered after our session was over.

I am very much looking forward to your upcoming workshop! Anyone who is interested in understanding what is going on in their body and what they need to balance it, NEEDS to make an appointment with you! What an incredible gift you have! Thank you!!!"
Jennifer Cummings/My Heart Reiki/Richardson, TX

"Having a food chart to assist me on my journey to optimal health and wellness, has made all the difference. While my focus was never on losing weight, it was a natural and effortless result of having and using my personal food chart. I look and feel better than I have in 20 years, and my energy, vitality and well-being are off the charts. I am so grateful for Gail and her gifts and the difference she is committed to making in the world. A forever grateful client."
Jen Smith/Waxahachie, TX

"I was fortunate enough to attend a 5 course dinner party for James Scott (President of Dallasvegan.com) made by Gail. Everything was delicious and it was obvious that care was taken in the choosing of ingredients for each course. You will feel nourished and satisfied with Chef Gail."
Christy Morgan /Author of Blissful Bites: Vegan Meals That Nourish Mind, Body, and Planet

"We recently had Gail at our office for a group cooking class. Her knowledge, passion, and energy are contagious. The food was amazing and can convert the worst eater to start getting some great natural, healthy food in their diet. She is an amazing resource for anyone that wants to naturally change their health and live a more energetic life."
Dr. James Fowler DC/Rowlett, TX

"Hey, Hey, Hey...Well all blood work and test are in and today I saw my doctor. NO DIABETES — clear! And, basically no thyroid issues either. By the way I went to the dentist about 2 weeks ago and she went to clean my teeth and she was so shocked that there was almost nothing to clean. She said a little bit of coffee stain. I don't drink coffee. The dentist came in and said don't know what you have done but this was great. Just had to tell you all the good news. You told me I was clear of the diabetes and in the four years with doctors and loosing almost 40 pounds I was never told I was clear. Your intuitive gift was such a life and game changer for me. I wasn't expecting the great dental report – Bonus! I don't mind at all you using this. My lab reports prove it."
Judy Kelley /Denton, TX

"Gail has helped me personally and my French Bulldog, Owen. I had a chronic yeast infection for the last four years, since I had my last daughter. And I had two toenails that were infected with fungus. I had tried everything to address the two. I have done Candida Cleanses, and treated with everything you can imagine—natural and traditional medicine. Gail has done for me in a few short weeks, what no other treatment could. I am now fungus free – internally and externally. For the first time in 10 years, my toe nails are growing back clear!

Owen is seven years old, and has had chronic yeast/fungal infections in his ears – to the point they are swollen and bleed. He also has had fungal infections on his skin. The vets would only prescribe meds that treat the symptoms. I bought every type of expensive, grain free food on the market, and we had no results. Enter Gail. With her intuitive skill, I'm able to know exactly what foods are compatible to Owen's bode. Within 2 weeks he was finally free of the infection! I can't say enough about Gail and how incredible she is. Thanks to her Owen can now live without constant irritation and itching. He's a happy dog again!"
Jessica Brown Wilson/Dallas, TX

"She isn't some mumbo jumbo chef to the stars that only makes dishes you can't pronounce with foods you've never heard of, or can't fix at home. She's raised 3 kids, she's from the "Real World", and has unlocked the SECRET to making healthy foods taste great, and can even do it on a shoe string budget."
Dr. Caleb Braddock /Van Alstyne, TX

"My session with Gail was fascinating and enlightening. She helped me narrow down a long list of foods to determine which ones would agree with my system. Eating those foods definitely felt great and it was such a relief not to be constantly wondering what to eat!!!"
Dr. Deb Kern/Austin, TX

"Gail's intuitive gift is amazing! She was able to pinpoint certain foods that my wife and I needed to avoid and other things that we need to be eating. Following her advice we are now seeing improvements in our health. Plus she shared great healthy recipes."
Pete Taboada/Visionary & Spiritual Artist

"About 6 months ago I was having some issues with my energy levels, sleep, and digestion and my thyroid was hurting which was causing me to worry. My lab test was positive for Hashimoto's. I was scared and I did not know how to treat this– and neither did anyone else. I found Gail through a friend and after following the food charts, I was feeling much better within a week. Knowing which foods to eat allowed my body to heal– my gut, my adrenals, and my thyroid. The fear is gone and I know how to take care of myself. Additionally, after taking a workshop with Gail last weekend, I know how to test myself for food compatibility. Food is medicine. Thank you Gail!"

Tanya Zolotnisky /Oakland, CA

Before We Get Started...

Quinoa is the "Star" of this book and I've already mentioned many of its healthful benefits. Did I mention it packs a whopping 8 grams of whole protein and 5 grams of fiber in 1 cup cooked? Being a seed, it naturally ranks very low on the glycemic index. This amazing super food can take the place of rice, hot breakfast cereals or add a protein boost to your smoothie. Oh, and it cooks in 15 minutes and freezes beautifully! It doesn't get much better than this!

Cook quinoa ahead and freeze in 2 ½ packed cup servings. Take quinoa out of freezer before you head to work. Many of these recipes you can make in a flash when this step is already done.

Basic cooking directions: Measure 1 cup of quinoa into a fine mesh strainer and place strainer into medium sauce pan. Fill pan with water and soak quinoa for 5 minutes. Drain water and rinse quinoa. Transfer quinoa back into pan with 2 cups of fresh water or broth. Bring to boil, reduce to low simmer, cover and cook quinoa for 15 minutes. Remove pan from heat and let stand for 5 minutes before uncovering and fluffing quinoa with a fork. 1 cup of dried quinoa makes 3 cups of packed cooked quinoa.

Note: For even easier digestion, use sprouted quinoa. True Roots is one brand or sprout your own. If using "sprouted" quinoa, reduce water or broth by half.

Avoid pesticides: Buy organic whenever possible. GMO (genetically modified organisms) foods are modified to resist damage from pesticides allowing more pesticides to be used.

The main GMO crops are corn, soy, canola and sugar beets (much of the granulated, non-organic sugar is produced from sugar beets now – not sugar cane). If buying organic is not within your budget, concentrate your organic dollars on the "dirty dozen" and what you eat the most. Go here for a list:

https://www.ewg.org/foodnews/summary.php

Keeping the balance: Adding a green salad to any meal is a great way to create healthy balance. I have included on page 24 and 25 a couple of easy and delicious alkalizing vinaigrettes for you to enjoy.

Note here: Many raw veggies and fruits may not be compatible with bodies that have stressed out digestive organs. The body has to do a lot of work to process raw food. Go easy on raw food until your digestion improves. Lightly steamed or roasted veggies may be better for you. The vinaigrettes are delicious on cooked veggies too.

Speaking of digestion: If raw foods are out for you, enzyme supplementation may be in order to aid digestion. We need enzymes for optimum digestion and they are abundant in raw fruits and veggies. Supplementation at meal time may help you get the most from your food until you can incorporate more fresh raw produce.

Nutritional Yeast is a magical food. It adds the rich, cheesy flavor to some of the recipes in this book. It is the "parmesan" in the "Italian Parmesan Vinaigrette" recipe below. Try adding this magic to soups, sprinkle on salads and veggies, etc. With about 5 grams of whole protein per 2 tablespoons and an excellent source of B-12, nutritional yeast has become a vegan's best friend! **Best part!**

It is neutral to slightly alkaline source of whole protein.

Note here: Nutritional yeast is grown on sugar beets and cane sugar (the label may not tell you which) so it is important to buy organic.

Ground Flaxseed is a super hero included in most of these recipes. 2 tablespoons equals 3 grams of whole protein and 5 grams of fiber. It is neutral in pH and ranks a big fat "0" on the glycemic scale. It lowers the glycemic load of any meal making it a diabetic's best friend. Enjoy it on oatmeal, sprinkle on yogurt and add to cornbread. I make an amazing vegan cornbread using ground flax in place of eggs. And, last but not least, flaxseed is a rich source of healthful, plant-based *omega 3 fatty acids.* Again, making it a vegan's best friend!

Note here: the "whole seed" is not digestible by most human bodies. Grind fresh to get the most benefit and store seeds or ground flax in freezer.

Coconut is Queen! Besides being luscious and delicious, lots of research now shows coconut oil and milk to be an extremely "brain healthy" food (rich in medium chain fatty acids the brain easily absorbs). Coconut oil also happens to be one of the few fats that are neutral to alkaline in pH. Cold-pressed olive oil is another very healthful neutral oil. Science is starting to show unrefined fat never was the enemy and is critical for health. Processed sugar is the real enemy. Read more here:
http://www.nytimes.com/2016/09/13/well/eat/how-the-sugar-industry-shifted-blame-to-fat.html

Speaking of coconut milk: I use organic So-Delicious

Unsweetened Coconut Milk Beverage in many recipes for its "non-descript" neutral flavor. This works well in savory recipes or when you do not want any sweetness. FYI - "Native Forest" brand organic canned coconut milk is clean and is stored in BPA free cans.

When I say "grass-fed" butter I mean butter from happy cows that are eating their natural diet of "GRASS". Kerrygold Irish butter is one brand I recommend.

About Stevia: You will notice I use Now Better Stevia Organic Liquid in many recipes to reduce sugar content. Much of the processed stevia on our grocery shelves (especially the powdered versions like Stevia in the Raw) are chemically processed and genetically modified (GMO) if not certified organic. Now is a brand I trust. The other is Nu Naturals Nustevia Reb99; however the powdered extracts are so sweet; I find it hard to get the amount just right in baking.

Miso is the secret ingredient that adds the rich, almost meaty flavor in many of my recipes. This is why my dad never misses the meat. I use dark miso (Eden Hacho) in tomato based sauces, soups and dark beans. I use sweet white miso (Miso Master) in white beans, lighter sauces and soups. Look for dark miso in the Asian section of your whole foods store and Miso Master in the refrigerated section next to tofu and vegan products. This fermented wonder is a powerful immunity booster with natural probiotic (good bacteria) that helps keep bad bacteria in check.

Speaking of fermented foods; all fermented foods provide the body with a healthy dose of good bacteria. Bragg's Unfiltered Apple Cider Vinegar is also a natural probiotic. And, helps detoxify and balance the body's pH.

I cook a lot in iron skillets. They are a GREAT source of iron for vegans. If you have old skillets lying around, break them out! My Dad's instructions for cleaning, seasoning and maintaining your iron skillet is at https://foodistalking.wordpress.com// (Look for Dad's Famous Cornbread Dressing Recipe. Instructions are at the end of the recipe).

Tapioca Flour is used to thicken sauces in some of these recipes. This super fine, white flour is gluten-free and tasteless. It can be used just like cornstarch and adds lightness to gluten-free baking.

Important note: tapioca and arrowroot will break down when too hot and the sauce will become thin. Remove the sauce from heat when it JUST starts to thicken. It will get thicker as it sits.

And lastly, I consider recipes to be templates. Feel free to substitute fruits, veggies and nuts as you desire.

Basic Alkalizing Vinaigrette   About 4 servings

3 tablespoons Bragg's apple cider vinegar*

1 tablespoon fresh lemon juice

2 tablespoons EVO (Extra Virgin olive oil)

2 teaspoons sweet white miso (Miso Master is my favorite)

1 teaspoon Dijon mustard

1 garlic clove, finely minced (optional)

1 teaspoon honey, maple syrup or a drop of liquid stevia (optional)

¼ teaspoon sea salt

Fresh ground pepper to taste

Blend all ingredients in a small processor or whisk together until smooth and creamy.

Remember, this is just the basic and IT IS amazing on its own. Try playing around with different spices, flavors and herbs. For instance; add fresh herbs like basil or cilantro. Or, create a spicy little number with curry powder and cayenne. Replace 1 tablespoon of Bragg's with sherry or balsamic vinegar for variety. Add a chunk of avocado for a creamy version (add water if too thick). Replace mustard, olive oil and 1 tablespoon of vinegar with 2 tablespoons of tahini. Let your imagination run wild!

Homemade Italian Parmesan Vinaigrette   8 - 10 Servings

½ cup Bragg's apple cider vinegar*

¼ cup organic extra virgin olive oil

2 garlic cloves, minced

1 teaspoon onion powder

¼ teaspoon dried red chili flakes (optional)

½ teaspoon dried oregano

½ teaspoon dried basil

2 tablespoons nutritional yeast

½ teaspoon sea salt and cracked pepper (or to taste)

Add all ingredients to a jar with tight fitting lid and shake well or process for a creamier version. This dressing will keep for a week to 10 days in the fridge.

For pennies per serving you have a fresh, chemical-free dressing that takes less than 5 minutes to make.

TIP: Always keep various vinegars, oils and spices on hand to whip up a quick dressing anytime! For instance; replace ½ of the Bragg's with red wine vinegar and omit nutritional yeast for red wine Italian vinaigrette.

*Note: (Bragg's raw vinegar is a natural, healthy probiotic and alkalizing to the body)

Chef Gail's Favorite Ingredients

Aroy-D Coconut milk
Better Than Bouillon Organic Vegetable Base
Bob's Red Mill Organic Grains and Flours
Bragg's Raw Apple Cider Vinegar
California Olive Ranch Olive Oil
Eden Hacho Miso
Imagine No Chicken Broth
Kerrygold Irish Butter
LeJoyva Instant Coffee
Lily's Sugar-Free Chocolate
Maple-Hill Creamery
Miso Master Sweet White Miso
Mezzeta Sugar Free Pasta Sauce
Native Forest Coconut Milk (BPA Free Cans)
Now Better Stevia organic liquid
Nustevia Reb 99
Parm Vegan Parmesan Cheese
Primal Kitchen Mayo
Rao's Homemade Pasta Sauce
Savoy Coconut Cream
So Delicious Coco Whip
So Delicious Coconut Milk Beverage, unsweetened
True Roots Organic Sprouted Quinoa
Wallaby Yogurt and Sour Cream
Whole Foods 365 Organic California Olive Oil

Where To Shop

Amazon Prime
Green Grocer
Kroger Signature Stores
Sprouts
Trader Joe's
Thrive Market Online
Whole Foods Market

Breakfasts, Desserts & Snacks

(Sometimes you just gotta have dessert first)

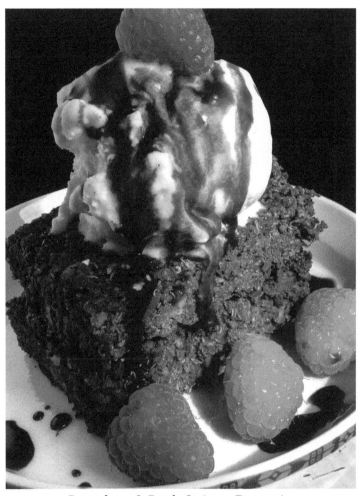

Decadent & Dark Quinoa Brownie

INDEX

Apple Crisp
Vegetarian/Vegan Option**   8 Servings

---

2 ½ cups cooked and cooled quinoa

4 tablespoons ground flaxseed + ½ cup water

⅓ cup full-fat coconut milk or other unsweetened, plant-based milk

2 tablespoons maple syrup (or 8 drops Now Better Stevia organic liquid)

1 teaspoon vanilla extract

½ teaspoon sea salt

Coconut oil or grass-fed butter

1. Preheat oven to 350ºF. Coat a 9 x 13 inch baking dish with a fine layer of coconut oil or butter.

2. In a large mixing bowl, whisk together flaxseed and water. Allow mixture to stand at room temperature until thickened to an "egg-like" consistency, about 5 minutes.

3. Whisk into flaxseed mixture; milk, syrup or stevia, vanilla and salt. Fold in quinoa and mix until thoroughly combined. Press quinoa mixture evenly and firmly into the bottom and slightly up sides of prepared baking dish. Bake for 15 minutes. Remove from oven and set aside.

Filling

4 firm tart apples peeled, cored and diced (Honey Crisp is my favorite)

1 teaspoon lemon juice

2 teaspoons cinnamon

½ teaspoon ground ginger

½ cup coconut palm sugar

1 cup rolled oats (Bob's Red Mill Organic is Gluten-Free)

1 cup oat flour

½ cup organic plain corn flakes, crushed

½ cup melted grass-fed butter (or coconut oil for vegan version)

½ cup chopped walnuts or pecans (optional)

1. Toss apples in lemon, spices and sugar. Spread apple mixture on top of baked quinoa.
2. Mix together balance of ingredients and spread evenly over apple mixture.
3. Bake for about 35 – 40 minutes or until apples are tender and bubbly.
4. Allow to cool for 10 minutes before slicing and serving. Perfect with a scoop of your favorite non-dairy vanilla ice cream – yum!

NOTE: Experiment with different fruit. For example; this would make a delicious Peach Cobbler!

Carrot Cake with Butter Cream Frosting
Vegetarian/Vegan Option   8-10 Servings

---

2 ½ cups cooked and cooled quinoa

4 tablespoons ground flaxseed + ½ cup water

⅓ cup full-fat canned coconut milk (or unsweetened, plant-based milk)

⅓ cup pure maple syrup or raw honey

8 drops Now Better Stevia organic liquid (or to taste)

1 teaspoon vanilla extract

2 teaspoons cinnamon

¼ teaspoon sea salt

1 cup shredded carrots

¼ cup raisins, dried currants or chopped dates (dates are low glycemic)

½ cup chopped walnuts or pecans (optional)

Coconut oil or grass-fed butter

1. Preheat oven to 350ºF. Coat 8 x 8 inch baking dish with a fine layer coconut oil or butter.

2. In a large mixing bowl, whisk together flaxseed and water. Allow mixture to stand at room temperature until thickened to an "egg-like" consistency, about 5 minutes.

3. Whisk into flaxseed mixture; milk, syrup or stevia, vanilla and spices. Stir in carrots, quinoa, raisins and nuts. Pour into prepared pan and spread evenly.

4. Bake for 35-40 minutes until set. A toothpick inserted should come out clean. Remove from oven and let cool completely before frosting.

Butter Cream Frosting

¼ cup unsalted butter, softened (Earth Balance Butter for vegan version)

½ cup cream cheese, softened (Tofutti cream cheese for vegan version)

¼ cup organic confectioners sugar (or ¼ teaspoon Now Better Stevia organic liquid, or to taste)

Splash of lemon juice

1 teaspoon vanilla extract

With an electric mixer beat the butter and cream cheese together until smooth and blended. Add stevia, lemon juice and vanilla. Whip until sugar is completely incorporated and frosting is very smooth and creamy. Or, just put it all in a food processor and process until creamy.

Cut room temperature or cold carrot cake into squares and serve with a big dollop of frosting and a few julienned carrots. Or, spread frosting on cake before slicing. In the picture I stacked 2 pieces and spread frosting between the layers for a traditional look.

Cinnamon French Toast
Vegetarian 8-10 Servings

---

2 ½ cups cooked and cooled quinoa

4 eggs, beaten, plus 1 uncracked

⅓ cup organic milk (or unsweetened, plant-based milk for non-dairy version)

⅓ cup maple syrup (or ¼ teaspoon Now Better Stevia organic liquid)

1 teaspoon vanilla extract

1 tablespoon cinnamon

Coconut oil spray

1. Preheat oven to 350ºF. Coat a 12 x 16 inch sheet pan with a fine layer of coconut oil. Whisk together eggs, milk, syrup or stevia, vanilla and cinnamon; then fold in quinoa. Press batter evenly and firmly into pan. Bake for 35 - 40 minutes or until just starting to brown around the edges. Remove from oven and cool completely.

2. Slice baked quinoa into 2 x 4 inch strips. **Note:** At this point you can freeze the quinoa for French toast or simply pop a slice in the toaster oven and serve with peanut butter, jam, etc. Just separate each slice with parchment to prevent them sticking together in freezer. **FYI –** Trader Joe's has fabulous no-sugar jams.

3. Heat a griddle over medium high. Whisk one egg until foamy and transfer to a shallow dish. Using a spatula to gently dip quinoa strip into egg and flip to coat both sides. Spray griddle with oil only where you will be dropping a slice. Dip, spray, drop, repeat. Toast quinoa for a couple of minutes on both sides or until egg is cooked and just starting to brown. Remove to plate and cover with foil to keep warm.

4. Serve with butter and warm pure maple syrup or honey. Try topping with sliced bananas and nuts with a sprinkle of cinnamon or nutmeg. Simple and Amazing!

Coffee Cake with Cinnamon Streusel
Vegetarian/Vegan Option 8 Servings

---

2 ½ cups cooked and cooled quinoa

4 eggs, beaten or 4 tablespoons ground flax seed + ½ cup water

⅓ cup unsweetened plant-based milk

⅓ cup honey (or ¼ teaspoon Now Better Stevia organic liquid)

1 teaspoon vanilla extract

Dash of sea salt

Coconut oil or grass-fed butter

1. Preheat oven to 350ºF. Coat a 9 x 13 inch glass baking dish with a fine layer of coconut oil or butter.

2. In a large mixing bowl, whisk together flaxseed and water. Allow mixture to stand at room temperature until thickened to an "egg-like" consistency, about 5 minutes. If using eggs; whisk until foamy.

3. Into eggs or flaxseed mixture; whisk in milk, honey or stevia, vanilla and salt. Fold in quinoa. Press quinoa mixture evenly and firmly into bottom and slightly up sides of prepared baking dish. Bake for 15 minutes and remove from oven.

Streusel

⅓ cup organic oat flour (Bob's Red Mill is Gluten-Free)

¼ cup cold grass-fed butter (or cold coconut oil for vegan version)

¼ cup coconut palm sugar (low glycemic)

1 tablespoon cinnamon

½ cup chopped walnuts or pecans

In a large mixing bowl, crumble oat flour and butter with a fork. Mix in coconut palm sugar and cinnamon. Fold in nuts.

Top baked quinoa with crumbled oat mixture. Bake for another 20 to 25 minutes or until topping is starting to brown. Remove from oven and cool completely before cutting.

Coffee break heaven!

Decadent & Dark Quinoa Brownies
Vegetarian/Vegan Option   10 Servings

---

2 ½ cups cooked and cooled quinoa (use black quinoa to fool those afraid of healthy)

4 tablespoons ground flax seed + ½ cup water

½ cup full-fat canned coconut milk

⅓ cup agave syrup (low glycemic)

¼ teaspoon Now Better Stevia organic liquid (or to taste)

⅓ cup organic unsweetened cocoa

¼ teaspoon instant coffee (my favorite is Le'Joyva)

Dash or 2 of chipotle or ancho chili pepper (optional – ever see the movie "Chocolat?")

¼ teaspoon sea salt

1 teaspoon vanilla extract

⅓ cup dark chocolate chips (Lily's is sweetened with stevia and amazing!)

½ cup chopped walnuts or pecans (optional)

Coconut oil or grass-fed butter

1. Preheat oven to 350ºF. Coat an 8 x 11 inch baking dish with a fine layer of coconut oil or butter.

2. In a large mixing bowl; whisk together flaxseed and water. Allow mixture to stand at room temperature until thickened to an "egg-like" consistency, about 5 minutes.

3. Into flaxseed mixture; whisk in everything except quinoa,

chocolate chips and nuts.

4. Fold quinoa into chocolate batter and combine well. Fold in nuts and chocolate chips. Pour batter into prepared dish and spread evenly.

5. Bake for 35 – 40 minutes or until completely set and toothpick comes out clean. Cool for 15 minutes before slicing.

Serve this chocolate decadence warm with coconut whipped cream; ice cream drizzled with chocolate sauce; or a dollop of the icing below. Heaven is biting into a gooey chocolate chip!

Chocolate Cream Icing

1 large avocado, smashed

⅓ cup cocoa (unsweetened)

⅓ cup agave nectar or honey

8 drops Now Better Stevia organic liquid for added sweetness (optional)

¼ teaspoon instant coffee (my favorite is Le'Joyva)

1 teaspoon vanilla extract

Dash of cinnamon

Dash of ground chipotle or ancho chili pepper (optional)

Dash of sea salt

Using a food processor, blend all ingredients until smooth and creamy. You can also do this with a hand-held mixer; just make sure you cream the avocado until very smooth before adding the other ingredients.

Sinful & Guiltless Dark Chocolate Sauce

1 cup full-fat canned coconut milk (or any unsweetened plant-based milk)

¼ cup coconut palm sugar

¼ teaspoon Now Better Stevia organic liquid, or to taste

¼ cup unsweetened cocoa powder

½ teaspoon instant coffee (my favorite is Le'Joyva)

¼ cup coconut oil or grass-fed butter

¼ cup Lily's chocolate chips

1 teaspoon vanilla extract

Dash of cinnamon

Dash of chipotle or ancho chili powder

½ teaspoon arrowroot or tapioca flour

Add all ingredients to a medium size sauce pan. Heat very gently while stirring often until chocolate and butter is melted. Bring to gentle simmer until smooth, creamy and JUST starting to thicken.

Note: The tapioca flour will break down when too hot and the sauce will become thin. Remove from heat immediately. Re-heat very gently to serve warm.

Homemade Coconut Whipped Cream

1 can of cold coconut cream (Savoy has no additives)

2 teaspoons honey (or 4 drops Now Better Stevia organic liquid for no-sugar version*)

1 teaspoon vanilla extract

Large chilled stainless bowl

Open can of coconut cream, drain off excess water and scoop cream into your cold bowl. Add honey or stevia and vanilla. With a hand held mixer or stand mixer, whip the cream until light and fluffy (processor works well too). Keep cold until ready to serve.

This deliciousness will keep for up to a week in the refrigerator or freeze the left-overs (re-process before serving). It probably won't last that long! I use what's left for my coffee...yummy!

Note: I always keep a can of coconut cream in the fridge.

In a hurry? So Delicious Coco Whip is a ready-made packaged, organic coconut whipped cream that is very low sugar. The package looks like Cool Whip and can be found in the freezer section of your whole foods store. It's really delicious, but does contain "natural additives".

*Tip: A little lemon zest neutralizes any bitter taste from stevia.

Jack Daniel's Banana No-Bread Pudding
Vegetarian/Vegan Option   8 Servings

---

2 ½ cups cooked and cooled quinoa

4 eggs, beaten or 4 tablespoons ground flax seed + ½ cup water

⅓ cup full-fat canned coconut milk (or other unsweetened, plant-based milk)

⅓ cup pure maple syrup (or ¼ teaspoon Now Better Stevia organic liquid)

4 large very ripe bananas, roughly smashed

⅓ cup raisins, currants or chopped dates (dates are low-glycemic)

2 teaspoons vanilla extract

2 teaspoons ground cinnamon or to taste

½ teaspoon sea salt

½ cup chopped walnuts (optional)

Coconut oil or grass-fed butter

1. Preheat oven to 350ºF. Grease an 8 x 8 inch baking dish with a fine layer of coconut oil or butter.

2. If using flax seed egg substitute: In a large mixing bowl, whisk together flaxseed and water. Allow mixture to stand at room temperature until thickened to an "egg-like" consistency, about 5 minutes. If using eggs: In large mixing bowl, whisk them until foamy.

3. Add all other ingredients except quinoa and nuts. Fold in quinoa and nuts and mix until thoroughly combined.

4. Pour batter into prepared baking dish and spread evenly. Bake 35 - 40 minutes. It's done with a toothpick inserted comes out clean. Remove from oven and let stand for 10 minutes before serving.

5. Cut pudding into large bite size pieces and place in serving bowls. Top with dairy-free ice cream (sugar-free option) and drizzle with warm Jack Daniels Caramel Cream sauce before serving.

Jack Daniel's Caramel Cream

½ cup full-fat coconut milk

¼ cup coconut palm sugar (low glycemic)

2 tablespoons pure maple syrup (or 8 drops Now Better Stevia organic liquid)

¼ cup Jack Daniel's or other good quality bourbon whisky

¼ cup fresh squeezed orange juice

Pinch of ground clove

1 tablespoon arrowroot or tapioca flour

In a small sauce pan, whisk together all ingredients. Bring sauce to gentle simmer. Cook for a minute or so until sugar is dissolved; sauce is smooth and JUST starting to thicken. Immediately remove from heat. It will continue to thicken. Gently re-heat before serving if needed.

Oatmeal Cookie Bar
Vegan   8 Servings

Quinoa Layer:

2 ½ cups cooked and cooled quinoa

4 tablespoons ground flaxseed + ½ cup water

⅓ cup full-fat canned coconut milk or other unsweetened, plant based milk

1 teaspoon vanilla extract

¼ cup maple syrup (or ¼ teaspoon Now Better Stevia organic liquid for no-sugar version)

½ teaspoon sea salt

Coconut oil or grass-fed butter

1. Preheat oven to 350ºF. Coat a 9 x 13 inch glass baking dish with a fine layer of coconut oil or butter.

2. In a large mixing bowl, whisk together flaxseed and water. Allow mixture to stand at room temperature until thickened to an "egg-like" consistency, about 5 minutes.

3. Into flax mixture; whisk in milk, maple syrup or stevia, vanilla and salt. Fold in quinoa. Press quinoa mixture evenly and firmly into bottom and slightly up sides of prepared baking dish.

4. Bake for 15 minutes. Remove from oven.

Cookie Layer:

2 large ripe bananas, smashed

1 teaspoon ground cinnamon

¼ cup maple syrup (or ¼ teaspoon Now Better Stevia organic liquid for no-sugar version)

¼ cup full-fat coconut milk or unsweetened, plant-based milk

1½ cup organic rolled oats (Bob's Red Mill is Certified Gluten-Free)

¼ cup raisins or chopped dates (dates are low glycemic)

¼ cup dark chocolate chips, optional (Lily's makes a fantastic sugar-free version)

1. Smash bananas until creamy. Whisk in cinnamon, syrup or stevia and milk. Fold in oats, raisins or dates and chocolate.

2. Spread cookie batter over quinoa. Bake 35 – 40 minutes or until top is browning. Remove from oven and cool completely before cutting into bars.

These bars are amazing on their own or with nut and seed butters. A perfect rib-sticking, satisfying way to start the day or a quick snack anytime. They freeze well; just wrap individually for a fast snack on the go!

Pumpkin No-Bread Pudding with Caramel Rum Cream

Vegetarian/Vegan Option   8 Servings

---

2 ½ cups cooked and cooled quinoa

4 eggs, beaten or 4 tablespoons ground flaxseed + ½ cup water

⅓ cup full-fat canned coconut milk

⅓ cup pure maple syrup or honey (or ¼ teaspoon Now Better Stevia organic liquid)

1 cup cooked pureed pumpkin (canned is fine)

1 teaspoon pumpkin spice

2 teaspoons vanilla extract

2 teaspoons cinnamon

¼ teaspoon ground clove

½ teaspoon sea salt

½ cup walnuts (optional)

Coconut oil or grass-fed butter

1. Preheat oven to 350ºF. Grease an 8 x 8 inch baking dish with a fine layer of coconut oil or butter.

2. If using flaxseed egg substitute: In a large mixing bowl, whisk together flaxseed and water. Allow mixture to stand at room temperature until thickened to an "egg-like" consistency, about 5 minutes. If using eggs: In large mixing bowl, whisk them until foamy.

3. Add all other ingredients except quinoa and nuts. Mix until thoroughly combined.

4. Fold prepared quinoa and nuts into egg/pumpkin mixture and combine well. Pour batter into prepared baking dish and spread evenly.

5. Bake 35 - 40 minutes. Remove from oven and let stand for 10 minutes. Cut pudding into large bite size pieces and place in serving bowls. Drizzle with warm caramel rum cream before serving.

Caramel Rum Cream

½ cup full-fat coconut milk

2 tablespoons coconut palm sugar (low glycemic)

¼ cup pure maple syrup (or ¼ teaspoon Now Better Stevia organic liquid)

¼ cup dark rum or spiced rum

¼ cup fresh squeezed orange juice

Pinch of ground clove

1 tablespoon arrowroot or tapioca flour

In a small sauce pan, whisk together all ingredients. Bring sauce to low simmer. Cook until sugar is dissolved and sauce is smooth and JUST starting to thicken. Remove from heat immediately. It will continue to thicken. Gently re-heat before serving if needed.

Note: Coconut palm sugar adds the delicate, caramel touch to this rich sauce.

More Serving Ideas for No-Bread Puddings and Cream Sauces:

These puddings can be sliced like bread when completely cooled and frozen in single slices. Just separate each slice with parchment. Toast lightly and smear with butter or coconut oil before serving.

Try the rich and creamy sauces over ice cream; on cakes or in your holiday coffee!

"All-In-One" Lunch or Dinner

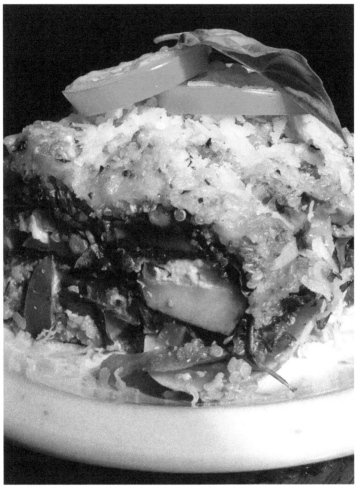

Kristen's Mediterranean Lasagna Casserole

INDEX

Butternut Squash, Collard & Portobello Bake
Vegetarian/Vegan Option   8 -10 Servings

Quinoa Layer:

2 ½ cups cooked and cooled quinoa

4 tablespoons ground flaxseed + ½ cup water

⅓ cup organic milk (So Delicious unsweetened coconut milk beverage for vegan version)

½ teaspoon sea salt

Coconut oil or grass-fed butter

1. Preheat oven to 350ºF. Coat a 9 x 13 inch glass baking dish or 4 quart casserole with a fine layer of coconut oil or butter.

2. In a large mixing bowl; whisk together flaxseed and water. Allow mixture to stand at room temperature until thickened to an "egg-like" consistency, about 5 minutes.

3. Into flaxseed mixture; whisk in milk and salt. Fold in quinoa. Press quinoa mixture evenly and firmly into bottom and slightly up sides of prepared baking dish. Set aside while you make the filling.

Squash, Collard, Mushroom Layer:

3 tablespoons butter (or olive oil for vegan version)

3 leeks, dark green tops remove, trimmed, washed and sliced thin (See video link on page 56)

3 garlic cloves, minced

2 cups roughly chopped Portobello mushrooms

3 tablespoons fresh chopped sage (or 1½ tablespoons dry rubbed sage)

1 teaspoon fresh chopped rosemary (or ½ teaspoon dried)

2 tablespoons tapioca flour

1 cup organic milk (So Delicious Coconut Milk Beverage, unsweetened for vegan version)

1 cup vegetable broth (Better Than Bouillon organic vegetable concentrate is great!)

2 tablespoons organic nutritional yeast

2 teaspoons sweet white miso (Miso Master is my favorite)

Sea salt and cracked pepper to taste

3 cups fresh chopped collard greens

2 cups cooked butternut squash, cubed (see directions on page 56 for baking whole squash)

Note: Kale and sweet potato can replace collard greens and squash

1. Heat deep large skillet or Dutch oven over medium high and add butter or olive oil. Add leeks and a fat pinch of salt. Sauté leeks for about 5 minutes. Add mushrooms, garlic, sage and rosemary. Sauté for another 3 minutes (keep it moving).

2. Sprinkle mixture with flour and stir to lightly toast flour for a few seconds. DO NOT BURN. Mix together the broth, milk and nutritional yeast. Gradually stir mixture into skillet. Continue to stir until sauce is JUST starting to thicken, 1 – 2 minutes. Remove from heat immediately.

3. Place miso into a fine mesh strainer and immerse strainer into sauce. With a wooden spoon dissolve miso into sauce. Stir mixture until miso is incorporated. Taste sauce for seasoning adjustments. Add salt and pepper if needed. Remove from heat.

4. Gently fold in collards and cubed squash. Pour mixture evenly over quinoa layer. Bake 35 – 40 minutes or until bubbly and browning around the edges. Remove from oven and let cool for 15 minutes before serving. Cut into squares and garnish with a fresh sage leaf or rosemary sprig.

For the vegetarian try a little melted asiago on top. The perfect rib-sticking, belly warming fall comfort food!

Baking directions for any winter squash: Preheat oven to 400ºF. Cut squash in half and remove pulp and seeds. Rub flesh with a little olive oil. Add a generous sprinkle of salt, cracked pepper and a pinch of nutmeg if you want. Place squash flesh side down on a foil or parchment lined sheet pan. Bake squash for about 20 minutes or until just tender but firm. When cool enough to handle, slice off skin and cut in to small cubes. **Note:** This freezes well for use later.

How to prepare leeks for cooking:
http://www.realsimple.com/food-recipes/cooking-tips-techniques/preparation/prepare-leeks

Tamale Pie
Vegetarian/Vegan Option   8 -10 Servings

Quinoa Layer:

2 ½ cups cooked and cooled quinoa

4 tablespoons ground flaxseed + ½ cup water

⅓ cup organic milk (So Delicious unsweetened coconut milk beverage for vegan version)

½ teaspoon sea salt

Coconut oil or grass-fed butter

1. Preheat oven to 350ºF. Coat a 9 x 13 inch glass baking dish or 4 quart casserole with a fine layer of coconut oil or butter.

2. In a large mixing bowl; whisk together flaxseed and water. Allow mixture to stand at room temperature until thickened to an "egg-like" consistency, about 5 minutes.

3. Into flaxseed mixture; whisk in milk and salt. Fold in quinoa. Press quinoa mixture evenly and firmly into bottom and slightly up sides of prepared baking dish. Set aside while you make the filling.

Filling:

2 tablespoons EVO

1 small onion, chopped

3 cloves of garlic, minced

1 yellow squash or zucchini, roughly chopped

1 ½ tablespoons chili powder

1½ teaspoons ground cumin

2 chipotle peppers in adobe sauce, chopped (or less for milder version)

1 cup cooked kidney or black beans, or a combo

1 cup organic whole kernel corn

14.5 ounce can fire roasted tomatoes

2 cups finely chopped fresh spinach

1 tablespoon dark miso, optional (I love Eden Hacho)

¼ cup fresh chopped cilantro, optional

1 teaspoon sea salt or to taste

Cracked pepper to taste

Tamale Layer:

3 tablespoons grass-fed butter (Earth Balance for vegan version)

1½ cups water

1½ cup full-fat organic milk (or lite canned coconut milk for vegan version)

1 teaspoon Bragg's Apple Cider Vinegar

1 tablespoon pure maple syrup (or 4 drops Better Stevia organic liquid)

1 ½ teaspoons sea salt

1 cup organic polenta (corn grits)

¼ teaspoon smoked paprika

1. Heat large pot or Dutch oven (iron is great!) to medium high. Add EVO and swirl to coat skillet. Add onion with a fat pinch of salt and sauté for 1 minute. Add garlic and squash. Sauté for another 3 minutes.

2. Add everything except cilantro, miso, salt and pepper and simmer veggies for about 10 minutes, stirring occasionally. Turn off heat. Add miso to a fine mesh strainer and with a wooden spoon dissolve miso into sauce. Blend well. Stir in cilantro. Add salt and pepper to taste. Set aside.

3. In a large sauce pan, melt butter. Whisk in all tamale layer ingredients and bring mixture to very gentle simmer. Cook for about 5 minutes, stirring constantly until polenta is very thick, but pourable, creamy and smooth.

4. Putting it together: Spread filling evenly on top of quinoa layer. Then spread tamale layer evenly on top of filling layer. Sprinkle casserole with smoked paprika and bake for 30 - 35 minutes.

5. Allow to cool for about 15 minutes before cutting into squares. Serve with a dollop of sour cream and fresh chopped scallions or cilantro with sliced avocado on the side.

Pot Luck Star!

Collards & Artichoke Bake
Vegetarian/Vegan Option   8 -10 Servings

Quinoa Layer:

2 ½ cups cooked and cooled quinoa

4 eggs, beaten or 4 tablespoons ground flaxseed + ½ cup water

⅓ cup organic milk (So Delicious unsweetened coconut milk beverage for vegan version)

½ teaspoon sea salt

Coconut oil or grass-fed butter

1. Preheat oven to 350ºF. Coat a 9 x 13 inch glass baking dish or 4 quart casserole with a fine layer of coconut oil or butter.

2. In a large mixing bowl; whisk together flaxseed and water. Allow mixture to stand at room temperature until thickened to an "egg-like" consistency, about 5 minutes. If using eggs; whisk until foamy.

3. Into flaxseed mixture or eggs; whisk in milk and salt. Fold in quinoa. Press quinoa mixture firmly into bottom and slightly up sides of prepared baking dish. Set aside while you make the next layer.

Collard and Artichoke Layer:

½ cup organic sour cream (Wallaby is grass-fed)

½ cup organic full-fat Greek yogurt (Wallaby)

¼ cup organic mayo (Primal Kitchen is clean and sugar-free)

3-4 garlic cloves, minced

⅛ teaspoon ground nutmeg

¼ teaspoon ground cayenne (optional)

1 teaspoon sea salt or to taste

1 teaspoon fresh ground black pepper or to taste

4 cups frozen chopped collard greens (thawed)

1 ½ cup chopped artichokes (packed in water and drained)

1 cup fresh grated parmesan or asiago, divided

1. In large mixing bowl, whisk together, sour cream, yogurt, mayo, garlic and spices.

2. Fold in collards, artichokes and ½ the cheese. Spread mixture evenly over quinoa and bake 40-45 minutes covered. Uncover, sprinkle top with remaining cheese and melt.

3. Allow to cool for 10 minutes before cutting into squares and serving.

Inspired by Food Babe, this creation is a healthy spin on a traditional party favorite!

For vegan option: Fold collards, artichokes, garlic and nutmeg into Béchamel sauce (see page 67 for recipe). Spread mixture on top of quinoa and bake as above. Top with vegan parmesan if desired. Parma is great!

Kristen's Mediterranean Lasagna Casserole

Vegetarian/Vegan Option   8 -10 Servings

---

*3 ¼ cups cooked and cooled quinoa, **(reserve ¾ cup)***

4 tablespoons ground flaxseed + ½ cup water

⅓ cup organic milk (So Delicious unsweetened coconut milk beverage for vegan version)

¼ cup nutritional yeast

½ teaspoon sea salt

Extra virgin olive oil

1. Preheat oven to 400ºF. Grease 9 x 13 baking dish with olive oil.

2. In a large mixing bowl; whisk together flaxseed and water. Allow mixture to stand at room temperature until thickened to an "egg-like" consistency, about 5 minutes.

3. Into flaxseed mixture; whisk in milk, nutritional yeast and salt. Fold in 2 ½ cups quinoa. Press quinoa mixture evenly and firmly into bottom and slightly up sides of prepared baking dish. Set aside while you make the filling.

Roast Veggie Layer:

1 tablespoon EVO

1 teaspoon garlic sea salt

1 large zucchini, cubed

1 large yellow squash, cubed

1 large red onion, roughly chopped

1 large red bell pepper, seeds removed and roughly chopped

Cracked pepper to taste

Marinara:

3 tablespoons EVO

1 small yellow onion, diced

4-6 garlic cloves, minced

2 cups sliced mushrooms (optional)

½ teaspoon fennel seed (optional)

1 teaspoon dried oregano

½ teaspoon dried basil

½ teaspoon red pepper flakes (optional)

¼ cup sliced Kalamata olives (optional)

24 ounce jar of marinara sauce, no added sugar (Mezzetta or Rao's Homemade)

1 tablespoon Eden Hacho miso, optional

Sea salt and cracked pepper to taste

Cheese Filling/Spinach and Basil Layer:

1 cup full-fat cottage cheese*

½ cup organic goat cheese or feta*

2 cups fresh packed spinach leaves

½ cup fresh chopped basil leaves

Topping:

¼ cup nutritional yeast

¾ cup cooked quinoa

½ cup shredded cheese Italian blend*

1 egg* (look for "organic pasture raised" – Vital Farms is one brand)

In a very large mixing bowl, whisk together 1 tablespoon olive oil and garlic salt. Toss in zucchini, squash, yellow onion and bell pepper. Continue to toss until veggies are evenly coated with seasoned oil. Turn out into large sheet pan and sprinkle with cracked pepper to taste. Roast veggies for about 20 minutes while preparing other layers.

1. Preheat large stainless or iron skillet over medium high. Add 3 tablespoons olive oil. Swirl to coat skillet and add onions with fat pinch of salt. Sauté for 3 minutes. Reduce heat to medium. Add to skillet; garlic, fennel, dried herbs, red pepper flakes and mushrooms (in that order). Continue to sauté for another 3 minutes.

2. Add olives and marinara. Simmer sauce for 10 minutes, stirring occasionally. Turn off heat. Add miso to a fine mesh strainer and with a wooden spoon dissolve miso into sauce. Blend well. Taste and adjust seasoning. Set aside.

3. In mixing bowl (or processor) blend together cottage cheese and goat cheese. Set aside.

4. In another mixing bowl, whisk egg and nutritional yeast together. Fold in ¾ cup quinoa and shredded cheese.

Putting it all together:

1. Spread ½ cup of marinara on top of prepared quinoa layer. Spread cottage cheese mixture on top of marinara. Arrange spinach and basil evenly on top of cheese. Top cheese evenly with 1 cup of marinara followed by roast veggies (press down veggies if need be to make more room). Spread the rest of marinara generously over veggies.

2. Lastly, evenly top casserole with quinoa/cheese mixture. **Reduce oven to 350ºF.** Tent casserole with foil and bake 20 minutes. Remove foil and bake another 20 minutes or until top is starting to brown around the edges and sauce is bubbly. Remove and let cool for 20 minutes before serving.

3. Garnish with fresh grated parmesan and a fresh basil leaf.

Lasagna is always a lot of work and this one is no exception. It is worth it – I promise!

*Vegan Option:

Vegan Ricotta Cheese

1 package of firm organic tofu

2 tablespoons fresh basil

½ teaspoon dried oregano

¼ teaspoon garlic powder

½ teaspoon sea salt

Dash of cayenne

¼ cup nutritional yeast

Drain all excess water from tofu and wrap in clean towel. Set aside to dry for a few minutes.

Roughly break up tofu and add to processor along with all other ingredients. Pulse in food processor until blended, but not smooth (ricotta like). Set aside in refrigerator. (You can mix this by hand - literally)

Vegan Béchamel Sauce: (Replaces Topping)

¼ cup Earth Balance butter

¼ cup of tapioca flour

2 cups So Delicious unsweetened coconut milk beverage, heated

¼ cup nutritional yeast

1 teaspoon Dijon mustard

½ teaspoon sea salt

½ teaspoon white pepper

1. In large skillet melt butter over medium high heat. Add flour and stir constantly for a minute until a smooth roux (thick paste) is formed (do not burn).

2. Add milk gradually while stirring constantly. Add nutritional yeast, Dijon, salt and pepper. Bring to gentle simmer and cook while stirring constantly until JUST starting to thicken. Remove from heat immediately. The sauce will continue to thicken. You should end up with a gravy-like, pourable sauce. Reheat very gently if needed.

3. Pour béchamel sauce evenly over roast veggies and bake as instructed.

Try this over broiled asparagus or pasta!

Savory Broccoli & Mushroom Casserole
Vegetarian/Vegan Option** 8 -10 Servings

Quinoa Layer:

2 ½ cups cooked and cooled quinoa

4 tablespoons ground flaxseed + ½ cup water

⅓ cup organic milk (So-Delicious unsweetened coconut milk beverage for vegan version)

½ teaspoon sea salt

Coconut oil or grass-fed butter

1. Preheat oven to 350ºF. Coat a 9 x 13 inch glass baking dish or 4 quart casserole with a fine layer of coconut oil or butter.

2. In a large mixing bowl; whisk together flaxseed and water. Allow mixture to stand at room temperature until thickened to an "egg-like" consistency, about 5 minutes.

3. Into flaxseed mixture; whisk in milk and salt. Fold in quinoa. Press quinoa mixture evenly and firmly into bottom and slightly up sides of prepared baking dish. Set aside while you make the filling.

Filling:

1 pound fresh chopped broccoli with stems, lightly steamed (or 3 cups frozen, thawed)

2 tablespoons grass-fed butter (EVO for vegan version)

1 tablespoon EVO

2 large leeks trimmed, washed well and chopped (or 1 large sweet onion)

2 large celery stalks, chopped

3 garlic cloves, minced

1 teaspoon dried thyme

2 cups chopped mushrooms (cremini or baby bellos are best)

⅓ cup nutritional yeast

2 cups organic milk (So Delicious unsweetened coconut milk beverage for vegan version)

2 tablespoons tapioca flour or arrowroot

1 ½ teaspoons sea salt or to taste

Cracked pepper to taste

1. In large, deep stainless or iron skillet, melt butter over medium high heat. Add olive oil, onions and celery with a fat pinch of salt. Sauté for a few minutes and then add garlic, thyme and mushrooms. Continue to sauté for about 5 more minutes.

2. Whisk together; nutritional yeast, milk and flour. Pour over mushroom mixture and simmer until sauce is JUST starting to thicken. Remove skillet from heat immediately.

3. Fold broccoli into mushroom sauce. Spread mixture evenly over quinoa layer. Bake 35-40 minutes. Allow to cool for 10 minutes before serving.

Sides or Main Event

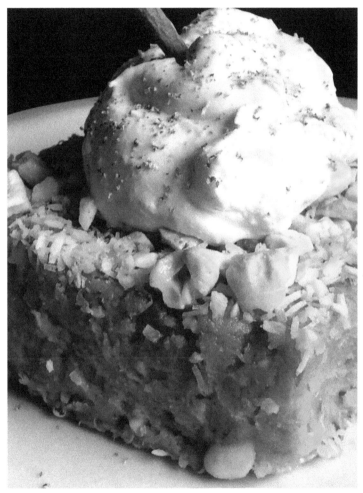

Yummy Yam Bake

INDEX

Apple, Cranberry & Sage Bake

Vegetarian/Vegan Option   8 -10 Servings

---

2 ½ cups cooked and cooled quinoa

4 tablespoons ground flaxseed + ½ cup water

⅓ cup organic milk (So Delicious unsweetened coconut milk beverage for vegan version)

Coconut oil or grass-fed butter

1. Preheat oven to 350ºF. Coat a 9 x 13 inch glass baking dish with a fine layer of coconut oil or butter.

2. In a large mixing bowl; whisk together flaxseed and water. Allow mixture to stand at room temperature until thickened to an "egg-like" consistency, about 5 minutes.

3. Into flaxseed mixture; whisk in milk and salt. Fold in quinoa. Press quinoa mixture evenly and firmly into bottom and slightly up sides of prepared baking dish. Set aside while you make the filling.

Filling:

2 cups fresh cranberries

½ cup honey (or ½ teaspoon Now Better Stevia organic liquid for no-sugar version)

½ cup water (add ½ cup if using stevia)

¼ teaspoon cardamom

½ teaspoon cinnamon

1 tablespoon fresh minced sage

1 teaspoon lemon juice and ½ teaspoon lemon zest

4 large Honey Crisp apples, cored and sliced thin (Fuji or McIntosh will do)

Homemade coconut whipped cream (see page 43)

Fresh sage leaves for garnish

1. In large pot; add cranberries, honey or stevia, water, cardamom and cinnamon. Bring to simmer and cook for about 5 minutes. Remove from heat and stir in sage, lemon juice and zest. Fold in apples.

2. Spread apple cranberry mixture over quinoa and bake 35 - 40 minutes or until quinoa is set and topping is bubbly. Remove from oven and let cool for about 15 minutes before serving. Slice and serve with a dollop of whipped cream. Garnish with fresh sage leaf.

Beautiful for dessert, breakfast or at your holiday table!

Broccoli & Cheddar Bake
Vegetarian/Vegan Option   8 -10 Servings

Quinoa Layer:

2 ½ cups cooked and cooled quinoa

4 tablespoons ground flaxseed + ½ cup water

⅓ cup organic milk (So-Delicious unsweetened coconut milk beverage for vegan version)

¼ cup nutritional yeast

½ teaspoon sea salt

EVO or grass-fed butter

1. Preheat oven to 350ºF. Coat a 9 x 13 inch glass baking dish or 4 quart casserole with a fine layer of EVO or butter.

2. In a large mixing bowl; whisk together flaxseed and water. Allow mixture to stand at room temperature until thickened to an "egg-like" consistency, about 5 minutes.

3. Into flaxseed mixture; whisk in milk, nutritional yeast and salt. Fold in quinoa. Press quinoa mixture firmly into bottom and slightly up sides of prepared baking dish. Set aside while you prepare the filling.

Broccoli & Cheddar Layer:

4 eggs*

1 cup organic milk*

1 teaspoon sea salt

Cracked black pepper to taste

1 ½ cup organic grated, sharp cheddar cheese, divided*

4 cups frozen broccoli florets, thawed

4-6 green onions, sliced thin on diagonal

1. In large bowl; whisk together eggs, milk, salt and pepper. Fold in 1 cup of cheese. Add broccoli and green onions to mixture. Stir until all is blended.

2. Pour the broccoli mixture over quinoa layer. Bake 35 – 40 minutes or until set and bubbly on top. Top with balance of cheese. Allow to cool for about 10 minutes before slicing and serving.

*Vegan Version:

In broccoli & cheddar layer; replace eggs, milk and cheese with the following:

3 cups unsweetened So Delicious Coconut milk Beverage

⅓ cup nutritional yeast

3 tablespoons tapioca flour

1 teaspoon Bragg's apple cider vinegar

½ teaspoon Dijon mustard

1 teaspoon sea salt

¼ teaspoon white pepper

1 teaspoon onion powder

½ teaspoon garlic powder

½ teaspoon smoked paprika

1. Whisk together all ingredients and pour into sauce pan. Bring to simmer and stir until JUST starting to thicken (1 or 2 minutes). Remove from heat immediately.

2. Mix sauce with broccoli and onions and spread evenly on top of quinoa layer. Bake as above. **Option:** Top with organic vegan shredded cheese and put back in oven for a minute to melt. Or, sprinkle with "Parm" Vegan parmesan.

TIP: For the best Vegan Mac & Cheese pour the sauce over cooked quinoa pasta shells (I like Ancient Harvest) and bake until bubbly. Top with organic vegan shredded cheese if desired.

Cheesy Roast Cauliflower & Caramelized Onion Bake

Vegetarian/Vegan Option   8 -10 Servings

Quinoa Layer

2 ½ cups cooked and cooled quinoa

4 tablespoons ground flaxseed + ½ cup water

⅓ cup organic milk (So Delicious unsweetened coconut milk beverage for vegan version)

¼ cup nutritional yeast

½ teaspoon sea salt

EVO or grass-fed butter

1. Preheat oven to 350ºF. Coat a 9 x 13 inch glass baking dish or 4 quart casserole with a fine layer EVO or butter.

2. In a large mixing bowl; whisk together flaxseed and water. Allow mixture to stand at room temperature until thickened to an "egg-like" consistency, about 5 minutes.

3. Into flaxseed mixture; whisk in milk, nutritional yeast and salt. Fold in quinoa. Press quinoa mixture firmly into bottom and slightly up sides of prepared baking dish. Set aside while you make the next layer.

Cauliflower and Onion Layer:

2 tablespoons EVO, divided

1 large head of cauliflower, cut into small florets

1 teaspoon garlic sea salt

2 tablespoons grass-fed butter

2 large sweet onions, cut in half and sliced thin

2 large eggs*

2 tablespoons Dijon mustard*

Pinch of fresh ground nutmeg

1 teaspoon sea salt*

½ teaspoon white pepper*

Dash of cayenne

1 – 8 ounce package chevre, softened (cream cheese or goat cheese will do)*

1 cup grated gruyere, reserve ¼ cup (Swiss will do)*

½ cup 2% organic grass-fed yogurt (Wallaby is good)*

1. Preheat oven to 400ºF. In large bowl; whisk together garlic salt and 1 tablespoon of EVO. Add cauliflower florets and toss until florets are evenly coated with oil. Spread cauliflower evenly onto large sheet pan. Sprinkle with cracked pepper to taste. Bake for about 20 minutes or until just starting to brown. Remove cauliflower from oven. Reduce heat to 350ºF.

2. While cauliflower is roasting, heat large skillet over medium high. Add 1 tablespoon EVO and butter. Swirl to coat pan. Add onions and a fat pinch of salt. Sauté onions for about 5 minutes

or until translucent. Reduce heat to medium. Cook, stirring occasionally to prevent sticking for about 20 minutes or until onions or nice and golden. Combine roast cauliflower with onions and remove skillet from heat.

3. In large bowl, whisk together eggs, Dijon, and spices. Fold in cheeses and yogurt (save ¼ cup gruyere!). Combine well. Mix in cauliflower and caramelized onions. Spread mixture on top of cooked quinoa layer and sprinkle with reserved gruyere.

4. Bake 35 - 40 minutes or until bubbly and browning around the edges. Tent with foil if starting to get too brown. Allow to cool for 15 minutes before serving.

5. Cut into squares and garnish with a little fresh chopped thyme or marjoram before serving.

*Vegan Option: See recipe on page 67 for Béchamel sauce that replaces cheeses, mustard, eggs, salt and white pepper (be sure and add the nutmeg to this).

Holiday Green Bean Casserole

Vegetarian/Vegan Option   8 -10 Servings

Quinoa Layer:

2 ½ cups cooked and cooled quinoa

4 tablespoons ground flaxseed + ½ cup water

⅓ cup organic milk (So-Delicious unsweetened coconut milk beverage for vegan version)

½ teaspoon sea salt

EVO or grass-fed butter

1. Preheat oven to 350ºF. Coat a 9 x 13 inch glass baking dish or 4 quart casserole with a fine layer of EVO or butter.

2. In a large mixing bowl; whisk together flaxseed and water. Allow mixture to stand at room temperature until thickened to an "egg-like" consistency, about 5 minutes.

3. Into flaxseed mixture; whisk in milk and salt. Fold in quinoa. Press quinoa mixture firmly into bottom and sides of prepared baking dish. Set aside while you make the green bean layer.

Green Bean Layer:

2 pounds of fresh green beans, trimmed and blanched (or 4 cups frozen and thawed)

3 tablespoons butter (Earth Balance Butter for vegan version)

2 cups sliced mushrooms (cremini or baby bellos are best)

¼ cup finely sliced shallots

3 garlic cloves, minced

½ teaspoon dried thyme

½ teaspoon dried marjoram

½ teaspoon white pepper

2 tablespoons tapioca flour or arrowroot

½ cup dry white wine (chardonnay is good)

1 cup vegetable broth (I love "Better than Bouillon Organic Vegetable Base in this)

2 tablespoons nutritional yeast

1 cup organic milk (So-Delicious unsweetened coconut milk beverage for vegan version)

Sea salt and cracked pepper to taste

1. Preheat oven to 375ºF. Bring 8 quart pan of water to rolling boil. Blanche green beans for 1 minute. Drain and place in ice water bath to stop cooking process. Set aside. (Skip this step if using frozen).

2. In same pan, melt butter over medium high heat. Add shallots and mushrooms with a fat pinch of salt. Sauté for a few minutes and then add garlic, thyme, marjoram and white pepper. Continue to sauté until mushrooms have released their moisture, about 5 more minutes.

3. Stir flour into skillet mixture, giving it a few turns (do not burn the flour!). Stir in wine and simmer for 1 minute.

4. Combine broth, nutritional yeast and milk and gradually add to pan stirring constantly. Add beans to mushroom mixture and

toss well to coat evenly.

5. Pour green bean and mushroom mixture on top of quinoa layer. Bake 35 to 40 minutes or until bubbly. Top with homemade Tabasco Onion Rings (recipe below)

Tabasco Onion Rings

1 very large sweet yellow onion (the flattest you can find or a Vidalia in season)

1 teaspoon Tabasco sauce

2 tablespoons tapioca flour

½ cup organic milk, (or So Delicious Coconut Milk Beverage, unsweetened)

½ cup tapioca flour

½ cup organic plain corn flakes (crushed)

¼ cup nutritional yeast

¼ teaspoon smoked paprika

½ teaspoon onion powder

½ teaspoon garlic powder

1 teaspoon sea salt

Coconut oil spray

1. Preheat oven to 450ºF. Spray large baking sheet with oil. Slice onion in ½ inch rings and separate. Set aside.

2. In small bowl, mix together Tabasco, 2 tablespoons flour and milk. Set aside.

3. Add the balance of ingredients to a paper or plastic bag (except coconut oil☺). Shake well to mix.

4. Submerge each onion ring in Tabasco batter and then place in bag. Shake to coat well. Remove and place on prepared sheet pan. Repeat with remaining rings. Lightly spray tops and sides of onion rings with oil before baking.

5. Bake for about 15 minutes or until rings are golden. Watch closely, all ovens are different. Serve immediately!

 A little work folks, but the best onion rings you will ever have – hands down! And, they are Gluten Free (no need to share this – no one will know). Don't make this casserole for your family this holiday season unless you are ready to bring it every year!

Sweet Corn Casserole

Vegetarian/Vegan Option   8 -10 Servings

Quinoa Layer:

2 ½ cups cooked and cooled quinoa

4 tablespoons ground flaxseed + ½ cup water

⅓ cup organic milk (unsweetened plant-based milk for vegan version)

2 tablespoons maple syrup

½ teaspoon sea salt

Coconut oil or grass-fed butter

1. Preheat oven to 350ºF. Coat a 9 x 13 inch glass baking dish or 4 quart casserole with a fine layer of coconut oil or butter.

2. In a large mixing bowl, whisk together flaxseed and water. Allow mixture to stand at room temperature until thickened to an "egg-like" consistency, about 5 minutes.

3. Into flax mixture; whisk in maple syrup or stevia and salt. Fold in quinoa. Press quinoa firmly into bottom and slightly up sides of baking dish. Set aside while you make the polenta layer.

Polenta Layer:

¼ cup grass-fed salted butter (Earth Balance for vegan version)

1 cup water

1 ½ cup buttermilk (or lite canned coconut milk and 1 teaspoon of

Bragg's vinegar)

¼ cup pure maple syrup (or ¼ teaspoon Now Better Stevia organic liquid)

1 ½ teaspoons sea salt (1 teaspoon if using buttermilk)

1 cup organic polenta (corn grits)

1 ½ cup organic whole kernel corn

¼ cup very thinly sliced scallions (green onions) - optional

¼ teaspoon smoked paprika (add a little chipotle powder for a little kick)

1. In a large sauce pan, melt butter. Whisk in all other ingredients **except corn, scallions and paprika.** Bring mixture to a very gentle simmer. Cook for about 5 minutes, stirring constantly until polenta is very thick put pourable. Remove from heat.

2. Spread whole kernel corn and scallions evenly over quinoa layer.

3. With a rubber spatula spread polenta on top of quinoa as evenly as possible. Sprinkle top with smoked paprika and bake 35 to 40 minutes.

4. Remove from oven and cool for 15 minutes before cutting.

Garnish with a dollop of sour cream and fresh chopped scallions or cilantro. I love it with fresh minced jalapeno and avocado. Or, make a chipotle sour cream (chipotle peppers in adobe sauce with sour cream – Oh man!). This will be the new favorite, holiday tradition!

No Turkey & Dressing
Vegetarian/Vegan Option   8 -10 Servings

---

2 ½ cups prepared white quinoa, (cooked with Imagine No Chicken Broth)

4 tablespoons ground flaxseed + ½ cup water

⅓ cup organic milk (So Delicious unsweetened coconut milk beverage for vegan version)

1 teaspoon Bragg's Apple Cider Vinegar

½ teaspoon sea salt

¼ cup nutritional yeast

EVO or grass-fed butter

1. Preheat oven to 350ºF. Coat a 9 x 13 inch glass baking dish or 4 quart casserole with a fine layer of EVO or butter.

2. In a large mixing bowl, whisk together flaxseed and water. Allow mixture to stand at room temperature until thickened to an "egg-like" consistency, about 5 minutes.

3. Into flax mixture; whisk in milk, vinegar, salt and nutritional yeast. Fold in quinoa. Set aside.

Next:

3 tablespoons butter (or Earth Balance butter)

1 large onion, chopped fine

2 large celery stalks, chopped fine

1 small red bell pepper, chopped fine

3 garlic cloves, minced

1 small apple, peeled and chopped fine

1 tablespoon rubbed sage (or to taste)

½ teaspoon dried thyme

½ teaspoon dried marjoram

½ teaspoon dried rosemary

1 cup Imagine No Chicken Broth

Sea salt and cracked pepper to taste

2 cups Beyond Meat Chicken Substitute (optional)

2 boiled eggs, chopped (or ¼ cup organic extra firm tofu chopped to look like boiled eggs)

1. Heat large stainless pot or Dutch oven (iron is great) over medium high and melt butter. Add onions, celery and bell pepper in that order with a fat pinch of salt. Sauté for 3 minutes. Add garlic and herbs, sautéing for another minute or until herbs are very fragrant.

2. Stir in broth and quinoa mixture. Add salt and pepper if needed to taste. Fold in meat substitute if using. Gently fold in boiled eggs or tofu. Pour dressing into prepared baking dish.

3. Bake for 35 to 40 minutes or until dressing is set (doesn't jiggle) and is starting to brown along the edges. Remove from oven and let cool for 15 minutes before serving.

Don't forget the cranberry sauce! There is a recipe on the back of every bag of fresh cranberries. Use ½ to1 teaspoon Now Better Stevia organic liquid for no-sugar version.

Yummy Yam Bake
Vegan   8 -10 Servings

---

2 ½ cups prepared quinoa, cooled

4 tablespoons ground flaxseed + ½ cup water

⅓ cup full-fat canned coconut milk

½ teaspoon sea salt

Coconut oil

1. Preheat oven to 350ºF. Coat a 9 x 13 inch glass baking dish or 4 quart casserole with a fine layer of coconut oil.

2. In a large mixing bowl; whisk together the ground flax and water. Allow mixture to stand at room temperature until thickened to an "egg-like" consistency, about 5 minutes.

3. Into flaxseed mixture; whisk in milk and salt. Fold in quinoa. Press quinoa mixture firmly into bottom and slightly up sides of prepared baking dish. Set aside while you make the next layer.

Sweet Potato Layer:

3 pounds of sweet potatoes, peeled and cubed

Water to boil potatoes

1 stick of cinnamon (about 2")

6 whole cloves

¼ cup cold-pressed coconut oil

½ cup full-fat coconut milk

¼ cup maple syrup (or ¼ teaspoon Now Better Stevia organic liquid)

½ teaspoon ground cinnamon (optional)

1 teaspoon sea salt or to taste

Topping:

½ cup cashews or walnuts

⅓ cup unsweetened flaked coconut

1. In large pan, add sweet potatoes, cinnamon stick, cloves and enough water to just cover potatoes. Bring to boil and reduce to simmer. Cook potatoes for about 15 minutes or until fork tender. Drain water and discard cloves and cinnamon.

2. In same pan combine sweet potatoes, coconut oil, milk, syrup or stevia, cinnamon and salt. Smash and stir mixture until desired consistency is reached (add a little more milk if you like a creamier texture). Spread mixture on top of quinoa layer.

3. Bake for 30 - 35 minutes. Add topping and bake for another 5 minutes or until topping is just started to brown. WATCH VERY CLOSELY! Coconut and cashews burn quick.

4. Remove from oven and let cool for 15 minutes before cutting into servings.

A dollop of coconut whipped cream takes the place of the marshmallow. Sprinkle with a little fresh grated nutmeg for an impressive presentation. This is super fantastic with pineapple as well! Just add chunks or rings on top of sweet potato layer before adding coconut and cashews.

Indian Spiced Version:

½ teaspoon fenugreek seed

1 red bell pepper, chopped

1 large shallot, minced

1 teaspoon ground coriander

¼ teaspoon ground cardamom

½ teaspoon white pepper

1. While potatoes are cooking, heat large skillet over medium high and add 1 tablespoon of coconut oil. Swirl to coat pan and reduce to medium. Add fenugreek seed and toast for a few seconds until fragrant. Add bell pepper and shallot. Sauté for about 5 minutes or until very soft. Add spices giving them a few turns to toast.

2. Stir mixture into smashed potatoes before spreading them on top of quinoa. Bake as instructed above.

All this flavor is worth a few minutes of extra time!

"Food _IS_ Talking" Chart of Foods

Here is the **Chart of Foods** designed for _"Food IS Talking"_ **Intuitive Food Compatibility Testing.** The pH of these foods have been tested intuitively. My answers may not completely agree with some of the answers you will find online. I have noticed that even the answers online vary from website to website. When used as a guide, the charts can help you create and maintain balance in the body. Most _"healthy and balanced"_ bodies can maintain an optimum pH by eating 60% alkaline and 40% acidic foods.

When the body is under any kind of stress (especially mental), it will need more alkaline foods. Stress creates acid in the body. The best thing you can do for your body is find ways to de-stress. I personally take long walks in nature, long baths and short meditations throughout the day (5 or 10 minutes).

I started meditating with "One Minute Meditation" (check it out here; https://www.youtube.com/watch?v=F6eFFCi12v8)
I would set the timer on my phone to go off on the hour to remind me to stop whatever I was doing; take a minute to breathe and disconnect from the world.   Anyone can do anything for one minute. I promise this practice will change your life!

Chart of Foods For *"Food IS Talking"* (Based on Organic Food)

Key: *Nightshade, **High Glycemic, X Extremely Alkaline, HA High Acidic, N Neutral, GF Gluten Free, ^Starches, HP High Protein

Alkalizing Vegetables

_Asparagus XHP
_Acorn Squash^
_Artichokes
_Beets
_Broccoli
_Butternut Squash^
_Brussels Sprouts
_Cabbage X
_Carrot
_Cauliflower
_Celery
_Collard Greens X
_Cucumber X
_Daikon
_Dandelion
_Eggplant*
_Fermented Veggies
_Garlic
_Green Beans
_Green Peas**
_Kale HP
_Kohlrabi
_Jicama X

_Leeks
_Lettuces X
_Mushrooms
_Mustard Greens
_Onions
_Parsley X
_Parsnips**
_Field Peas^
_Peppers (mild) *
_Hot Peppers
_Okra
_Potatoes**^**
_Pumpkin*^
_Radishes*
_Rutabaga
_Sea Veggies X
_Spaghetti Squash^
_Spinach XHP
_Sprouts
_Sweet Potato X^
_Swiss Chard XHP
_Turnip
_Zucchini*

Alkalizing Fruits

_Apples
_Apricots (_Dried**)
_Avocado
_Banana**
_Blueberries
_Blackberries
_Cantaloupe **
_Cherries
_Coconut
_Currants**
_Dates
_Figs**
_Grapes X
_Honeydew Melon**
_Kiwi
_Lemon X
_Lime
_Grapefruit
_Mango**
_Nectarine
_Papaya
_Peach
_Pear
_Raisins**
_Raspberries
_Rhubarb
_Strawberries
_Tomatoes *
_Watermelon X

Misc. Alkaline Items

_Almonds (raw) HP
_Almond Milk
_Apple Cider Vinegar X
_Coconut Milk
_Coconut Milk Ice Cream
_Honey X
_Sunflower Seeds (Raw)

Neutral and Acidifying Foods

Legumes/Beans/Veggie
(Legumes are Starch^)

__Black Beans **
__Black-eyed Peas
__Chick Peas HA HP
__Kidney Beans N HP
__Lentils N HP
__Lima Beans N HP
__Mung Beans N HP
__Navy Bean N HP
__Peanuts HA **HP
__Pinto Beans
__Red Beans N HP
__Spilt Peas HP
__Soy Beans HA HP

__Miso N HP
__Whole Corn HA ^
__Yellow Squash N

Nuts/Seeds

__Brazil Nuts N HP
__Cashews ^ HA
__Macadamias HP
__Pecans HP
__Pistachios HA
__Walnuts HP
__Chia Seed N
__Flax Seed N
__Hemp Seed HP
__Pumpkin Seeds N
__Sesame Seed N

Grains & Rice

__Amaranth ^ GF HP N
__Barley ^ HP
__Brown Rice **^ GF
__Brown Basmati**^GF
__Buckwheat ^ GF
__White Jasmine ^**GF
__Brown Jasmine ^** GF
__Kamut ^ N HP
__Millet ** ^ GF N
__Oat Bran ^ GF HA
__Quinoa N GF HP
__Rolled Oats ^ GF
__Rye ^
__Spelt ^ N
__Steel Cut Oats ^ GF
__Teff ^ GF N HP
__Wheat Germ ^**HA
__Wheat Bran ^**HA
__White Rice ^**GF
__White Basmati ^**GF
__Wild Rice ^ GF
__Wheat Berries ^ GF HP

Nut/Seed Butters

__Almond Butter N HP
__Cashew Butter ^HA
__Peanut Butter ^HP
__Sunflower Butter HP
__Tahini (Sesame)

Flours/Cornmeal

__Almond Flour N GF HP
__Bleached White^***HA
__Coconut Flour N GF
__Unbleach White^***HA
__Bean Flours ^GF HP
__Brown Rice Flour^***GF
__Oat Flour ^ GF
__Rye Flour ^ GF
__Sorghum ^***GF
__Whole Wheat^***HA
__Cornmeal^GF
__Polenta/Grits^GF
__Tapioca Flour ^GF
__Arrowroot ^ GF

Dairy/Eggs
(All HP)

__Cheddar Cheese HA
__Cottage Cheese N
__Goat Cheese
__Goat Feta
__Sheep Feta (French) N
__Gouda HA
__Mozzarella
__Parmesan HA
__Swiss
__Pasteurized Ice Cream HA
__Pasteurized Milk HA
__Raw Milk
__Kefir N (Buttermilk)
__Yogurt N
__Raw Milk Yogurt N
__Goat Milk N
__Eggs HA

Fruits

__ Fresh Cranberries HA
__Dried Cranberries**HA
__Orange**HA
__Pineapple **HA
__Plum
__Prunes**
__Tangerine**HA

Sugars/Substitutes

__Agave Syrup HA
__Black Strap Molasses
__Brown Rice Syrup**HA
__Brown Sugar**HA
__Coconut Palm Sugar
__Date Syrup
__Maple Syrup
__Pure Cane Sugar **HA
__Stevia (liquid)
__Xylitol (corn/birch Xyla)

Vinegars

__Balsamic HA
__Champagne
__Plum Vinegar
__Red Wine HA
__Rice HA
__Sherry Vinegar
__White Balsamic

__Kombucha **
__French Market Coffee

Oils

__Avocado Oil N
__Cold Pressed Coconut N
__Luanne Coconut
__Butter (grass fed) N
__Corn Oil HA
__Olive Oil N
__Peanut Oil
__Safflower Oil HA
__Sesame
__Walnut
__Grape seed oil
__Flaxseed oil N
__Spray Coconut oil

Nature Fed Meat/Poultry

__Venison HA
__Beef HA
__Bison HA
__Chicken HA
__Lamb
__Pork HA
__Processed Meats HA
__Turkey

Plant Milks

__Soy HA
__Rice **
__Coconut Beverage N
__Hemp (Manitoba) HP
__Quinoa milk HP
__Carrageenan
__Gaur Gum

Fish (Wild Caught)
(All HP)

__Catfish HA
__Cod
__Salmon
__Sardines
__Sea Bass
__Tilapia HA
__Tuna HA
__Halibut

Shellfish (Wild Caught)

__Clams HA
__Crab
__Lobster HA
__Scallops HA
__Shrimp HA
__Oysters

Misc. Acidifying Foods
(Most alcohol is not GF)

__Chocolate 70% HA
__Red Wine HA
__White Wine HA**
__White Liquors HA
__Brown Liquors HA
__Beer HA
__Egg Noodles HA**
__Rice Noodles HA**
__Nutritional Yeast N HP
__Hummus HA HP
__Black Tea HA/Green
__Coffee HA

What's Next

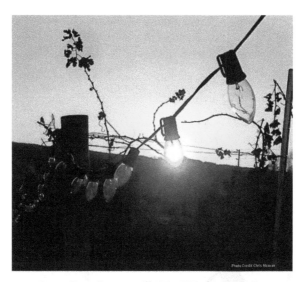

Evolution of FREE Health

"The 6 Missing Links to Abundant Health"

Without Our God-Given Health. We Are "Not Free"

The 6th Missing Link – "We are the commander of our vessel when we realize WE ARE. Each missing link "re-discovered" brings us closer and closer to freedom."

Intuitive Chef Gail Blair

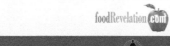

"Food _IS_ Talking" **The 10 Most Compatible Foods Cookbook**
What the Body Cannot Digest it Cannot Use.
What the Body Cannot Use Becomes a Burden.

Want to be notified when books are launched? Sign up for the foodRevelation.com newsletter; full of healthy inspiration and recipes! http://foodrevelation.com/

About the Chef

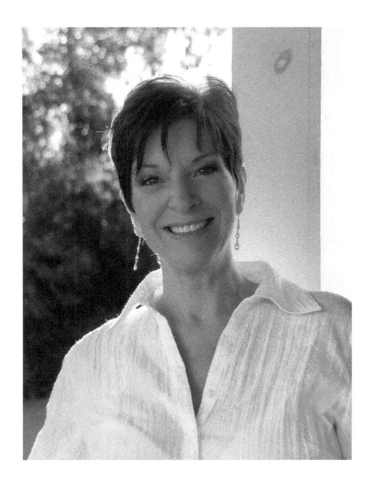

Gail's "Intuitive Chef" journey started unfolding in 2009 when she began "working" her passion creating delicious, nutritious food. foodRevelation.com and "Food *IS* Talking" are the natural result of following her creative passion. Gail now works full-time as a Food and Medical Intuitive helping clients all over the U.S. and Canada re-discover their God-given health and in-born intuition.

Gail lives with her beloved Pitbull mix Molly in a small town in North Texas. In addition to the joy of cooking and recipe creation, she finds great pleasure in long leisurely meals with family and friends, reading, writing; long quiet walks in nature and sleeping under the stars.

Keep up with Gail on Facebook at
https://www.facebook.com/foodrevelation/ and on Twitter at
https://twitter.com/foodrevelation and at
https://goodfood4thought.wordpress.com

Contact Gail at http://foodrevelation.com/contact-us/

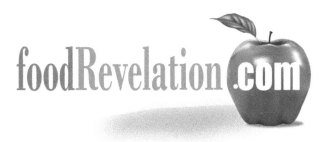

Our in-born intuition and the power of our thoughts can lead us to health and happiness. My passion is food. My mission:

"Empowering others to Empower Themselves"

CPSIA information can be obtained
at www.ICGtesting.com
Printed in the USA
LVHW01*0832151117
556358LV00005B/6/P